The Self-Empowering Sleep Book

DELBERT CURTIS

www.BooksForAChange.com

Disclaimer

This book details the author's personal experiences with, and opinions about, The Self-Empowering Sleep Book. The author is not a healthcare provider.

The author and publisher are providing this book and its contents on an "as-is" basis and make no representations or warranties of any kind with respect to this book or its contents. The author and publisher disclaim all such representations and warranties, including but not limited to warranties of merchantability and healthcare for a particular purpose. In addition, the author and publisher do not represent or warrant that the information accessible via this book is accurate, complete, or current.

The statements made about products and services have not been evaluated by the US Food and Drug Administration. They are not intended to diagnose, treat, cure, or prevent any condition or disease. Please consult with your own physician or healthcare specialist regarding the suggestions and recommendations made in this book.

Except as specifically stated in this book, neither the author nor publisher, nor any authors, contributors, or other representatives will be liable for damages arising out of or in connection with the use of this book. This is a comprehensive limitation of liability that applies to all damages of any kind, including (without limitation) compensatory; direct, indirect, or consequential damages; loss of data, income, or profit; loss of or damage to property; and claims of third parties.

You understand that this book is not intended as a substitute for consultation with a licensed healthcare practitioner such as your physician. Before you begin any healthcare program or change to your lifestyle in any way, you will consult your physician or another licensed healthcare practitioner to ensure that you are in good health and that the examples contained in this book will not harm you.

This book provides content related to physical and mental health issues. As such, the use of this book implies your acceptance of this disclaimer.

Discover the online community!

Official Website

Get access to free downloads, forums, and news:
http://www.booksforachange.com/

Twitter

Stay up to date with new articles: @SleepCounselor

#SleepKeys
#SleepCuts

Instagram

Find valuable advice and inspiration: @SleepCounselor

#SleepKeys
#SleepCuts

Contents

Introduction

FOR MORE THAN twenty years, I experienced nights of chronic insomnia, nights when I was much more awake at three o'clock in the morning than I was during the day. I know them well—these nights without sleep, the interminable wait where all we want is just to find a bit of rest, which guides our last hopes until dawn. How is it possible to be kept awake all night, and then finally as the sun rises, be given a few hours—or even minutes—of respite?

For many years now, I have been insomnia free. This has allowed me to profoundly change my rhythm of life. I am like you, I have experienced how difficult life with insomnia can be and thought it would never change. Upon reflection, this change was not as impossible as it seemed, and I am excited to share my experiences and techniques with you.

If you have chosen this book, it is almost certainly because we have shared the same experience. We have gone through similar difficulties, asked the same questions, known the same ordeal. I understand what it is like to wake up tired and still have to face your responsibilities. I experienced the struggle just to be present, to concentrate, and to cope with stress every day. I know how difficult it is not to let yourself be overwhelmed by the emotions that surface when fatigue is always present.

I tried everything: hot baths, herbal teas, going to bed early, pills, homeopathy. I refused, however, to try hormonal cures, preferring instead to train hundreds of flocks of sheep that could have excelled in the Olympic Games. I consulted specialists in many disciplines, but I never succeeded in solving my insomnia problem through their direction. I owe them my gratitude for their good advice and will pass on to you what I found most effective.

Too many years passed without finding solutions. I spent whole nights thinking, reflecting, trying to find answers and to figure out why. Why me? Why can't I fall asleep?

This is the book I wish I could have read back then.

I have been insomnia free for seven years. By designing a method, I was able to put an end to this unbearable rhythm. Now I can fall asleep regularly, without difficulty, calmly, just like everyone else. I know how to regulate my sleep rhythm, which allows me to be energetic, efficient in my work, and more fully present in all aspects of my life. Day after day, I can now develop the life I want: a healthy, sane, fulfilling one, free from the anxiety of waking up. The whole of my waking life has also greatly improved. How could it not?

I firmly believe in our individual ability to solve difficulties through our own will. This self-empowering way of thinking is especially true for sleep-related problems. It is possible simply through learning, self-observation, and the application of a clear step-by-step method. This is what you will find in this book.

※ ※ ※

In the United States, about 40 percent of the population (more than one in three people) sleep less than seven hours a night [1]. Lack of sleep has become a social problem. The average amount of nightly sleep has fallen from nine hours in 1910 to 6.8 hours per night [2]. This can be seen as a reflection of our hyperactive society, which aims for an ever-increasing amount of information and stimuli during the day. Today we have to deal with a world where it is increasingly difficult to disconnect, and therefore increasingly more difficult to *reconnect* with ourselves.

If you are reading this book, you are already on your way to a solution. For this, bravo! You have chosen change, and it is by seeking it that you find it. I truly hope this book is the last one you have to read on the subject.

Your journey and your difficulties are unique. There is no

easy, effortless way to do it. Permanent change always implies commitment. While there is no miracle tool, there are healthy tips that apply to everyone. There is also a step-by-step path to follow that you can be guided on. I am not a doctor, but like you, I am someone who has endured years of insomnia. Today, I am happy to have left them behind, to be able to publish what I have learned along the way, and to share the method I have developed.

I hadn't thought or planned to write a book about sleep, but after sharing this method with close friends, I saw how quickly their sleep improved. Thus, this book was born, with the hope that others may find the same relief.

※ ※ ※

There are many problems caused by a lack of sleep. Just to give you an idea, about 20 percent of road accidents in the United States are caused by drowsy driving [3]. In other words, the risks are not limited to a few bad nights.

To motivate one's commitment, it is good to observe the benefits that can be derived from it, not only in the immediate future but in the long term. Numerous studies show that a good night's sleep can reduce weight gain, reduce the risk of heart disease, Alzheimer's and high blood pressure, increase concentration, help find creative solutions, improve memory and mood stability, reduce the risk of type 2 diabetes, and improve libido in men [4].

All this is free and available to us. Need we say more to get started?

Who can you become once you have left insomnia behind? The answer to this question is reason enough to put all of your energy into change. And this change may not be so far away! Once the suffering of sleepless nights are gone, what can you unlock within? What life changes can occur?

The goal is to return to yourself, to become free and full of energy for yourself and, in turn, for others.

This book is intended to be as condensed as possible. It is not an inventory describing every sleep pathology. Though droning text could help knock you out in the short term, the aim of this book is to be practical, clear, and direct. It exists to pass on a method that can help you get to sleep quickly and, above all, sustainably. Welcome to change, here and now.

Chapter 1

Unraveling Change

EACH PATH IS different. Sleep problems have been a part of my life since I was a child. From the time I was born, I have always had very short nights, and consequently so did my parents. However, as early as the age of seven, I began to ask myself how I could fall asleep with more ease. By age eight, I had already developed the beginning of a solution. I would listen to my grandfather breathing as he slept and then try to match the slow rhythm of his breathing with my own. Simply increasing the length of each breath calmed me, and before I knew it, I would drift off to sleep. Although this technique was good, I quickly realized that it was no longer sufficient when the constraints of young adult life came to the forefront.

As with many teenagers, my sleep rhythm shifted, and the physical and mental capacity of my youth compensated for the state of sleep deprivation I encountered. Later, as an adult, the stress surrounding city life, work, and an accelerated pace of life quickly degraded the quality of my sleep even further. I often held study days and, later in life, workdays by the rhythm of three to five coffees per day to be able to meet my obligations. My quality of life was in decline. Not only was I maintaining this lifestyle at the expense of my health, but the quality of my work began to plummet, and my relationships suffered.

According to the Pennsylvania School of Medicine, 25 percent of the American population experiences insomnia every year [5]. Fortunately, in 75 percent of cases, people manage to recover without developing chronic problems. Unfortunately, this still leaves millions of people subject to insomnia, struggling with great difficulty and danger in their daily lives.

In the overactivity society demands, we find the

disappearance of our free time, flowing out of our lives toward the superfluous. Yet, it is precisely this personal time that is so precious and necessary for us to be anchored in ourselves. This is an invisible symptom of the acceleration of our times, and we must be able to reclaim it.

After this short presentation, I will leave my own experience aside as much as possible to describe only the learning that I think is most important and to present this simple, effective method.

The goal is to quickly improve your sleep and get you back to the life you want.

CHAPTER 2

Find the Origin—Touch the Solution

IN A STUDY conducted in France by INSERM (The National French Public Research Organization), 45 percent of twenty-five to forty-five-year-olds consider that they lack sleep. On average in France, the population sleeps one hour and thirty minutes less than it did fifty years ago. The change in sleep duration is a reality and a phenomenon that is widespread throughout the contemporary Western world.

There is no magic solution, but there are many habits that are healthy. We are all different and have to deal with different situations. Therefore, we must sincerely consider our individual psychological states.

Sleep loss does not happen all at once; it is a disorder that develops over time [6]. If you suffer from sleep disorders, it is very likely related to your lifestyle and/or concerns around personal life, family, or work. This may be due to anxiety produced by a change in your external environment (such as an external or environmental change in noise, light, etc.) or by an internal change (emotional, psychological, or disease related). It is, therefore, also central to reflect on the issues that are at the root of the problem.

For people suffering from conditions such as depression or other psychological disorders, it is essential to consult your doctor or a qualified specialist first. Though this book contains advice that can help you improve your nocturnal difficulties, it is also necessary to direct your efforts in the treatment of the underlying pathology in order to solve the fundamental questions.

Conventionally, insomnia is categorized according to its duration and whether it is related to another disease. When it is occasional and very disruptive, insomnia is often referred to as acute. When it is long term, we speak of chronic insomnia.

Types of Insomnia:

- **Primary**: When it applies to people whose sleep problems are not directly associated with other health problems.
- **Secondary**: When a person has sleep problems related to another cause. It could be associated with a health problem, for example: asthma, depression, arthritis, cancer. Somatic disorders such as heartburn, pain, or dependence on drugs or substances (such as alcohol) may be to blame as well.

Although the development of insomnia is gradual, it most often stems from the deregulation of our lives following an event. There can be many origins, such as intense stress (following the loss of a loved one, a job, a move); disorders due to anxiety, overwork, illness, and physical or mental pain; as well as problems due to the environment (noise, heat, or light). The use of certain medications or a change in your lifestyle (night work, jet lag) can also be contributing factors [7].

Recent research shows a strong link between the management of emotions and insomnia. Depending on the individual, this can cause more or less anxiety and stress. Insomnia can either be the consequence or the cause. For example, it can be the consequence of an emotional shock during a breakup, but perhaps the cause of disorders such as anxiety, something that affects about 24 to 36 percent of people with insomnia [8]. The relationship between the causes and consequences in each case is complex to identify, but what is known is that insomnia causes many physical and psychological disorders that feed our struggles.

Whatever disorder you are suffering from, healing begins when you sincerely accept that change via a step-by-step resolution is possible. The road is then paved day after day, and the focus of the journey shifts from speed toward change, to maintaining the right direction.

Why all this? Because there is one essential thing to

understand: there is no approach, no method that can solve the problem definitively for you simply by reading. You are the only one who has the opportunity to heal yourself, to put an end to the problem that initiated your insomnia.

How? By seeking to be at peace with yourself. By gradually moving toward the resolution of the problems that affect you.

We all know that things take time to settle. Through this book, we will start a journey together to allow you to improve your difficulties with insomnia. This is the beginning of a path, one you will naturally be able to continue on your own.

It is important to be able to find the help you may need around you. Consult your doctor, who will refer you to a specialist if necessary. This is all the more important for people suffering from secondary insomnia, linked to a disease or dependence. The advice and method described in this book will give you many tools that will become the keys to solutions, but it does not claim to, nor can it solve every trouble. There is no such magic cure.

Keep these two tips in mind:

- Though only you can make the road to change, you can be given precious indications about which road to follow.

- Change rarely happens in an instant; it is not a sudden and absolute realization, but a series of steps. It is the understanding of tests as well as small changes in one's daily life that will gradually and definitively solve each problem. This does not mean that the difficulty of the situation you are facing does not have an immediate resolution. On the contrary, you will be able to act immediately, but the complete resolution will take time and be more or less rapid depending on you and your situation. Change takes shape if it is decided and disciplined.

CHAPTER 3

BASIC ADJUSTMENTS

Technical Improvements

THERE ARE SEVERAL purely practical solutions that have often helped me find surprising improvements in sleep, for example, good soundproofing of your room. Simply finding calm during the night makes it possible to avoid waking up at odd hours or too early, thus eliminating any difficulties falling back to sleep. It also helps you to avoid any delays in falling asleep caused by external discomfort. However, soundproofing a room remains relatively complex and can be expensive. If it is a living space in which you know you will spend the next few years, then perhaps this option makes sense for you. Otherwise, there are other more immediate and cost-effective solutions, such as the use of earplugs, whose reputation to quickly restore silence is already well established. There are foam models with a noise reduction of about 35 dB and wax models with a reduction of 27 dB. However, depending on the sound frequency of a particular noise, some earplugs may be more effective than others. Some people prefer wax models because they can be perfectly adapted to the shape of the ear canal and therefore more impermeable to certain noises. (Be careful not to form a shape that is too elongated, or you may have difficulty removing them.)

However, these have one major defect: they can prevent you from hearing the alarm clock in the morning (especially if you are sleep deprived). And unless you set your alarm volume extremely high (which may inconvenience your partner or neighbors), you may sleep right through it.

There are then two solutions. One is the use of an alarm clock with natural light that gradually increases in brightness.

Using soft light and gentle tones to wake each morning is a much more pleasant experience than being jarred from sleep by harsh alarms. Starting each morning in this gentle way (especially if you experience anxiety upon rising) can be a simple trick to retrain your body, over time, to have a positive association to mornings.

The other solution is to fall asleep with comfortable headphones and quiet music. Headphones have their shortcomings, namely their instability on the ears. This has a certain advantage, though: it allows you to fall asleep with the headphones on, while natural nocturnal movements can cause them to fall off during the night. As a result, you no longer risk missing the alarm clock in the morning.

The temperature of the room where you sleep is important. The recommended temperature is 65° F (18° C). A room that is too hot or too cold can cause you difficulty falling asleep as well as increase the frequency of nightly awakenings. Also, it is important to avoid drinking too much water or herbal tea before going to sleep.

Over the seasons, your environment is subject to constant changes in humidity. Though it is recommended to humidify the air for infants, a humidity level between 40 and 60 percent is ideal for adults. You can find small indoor thermometers online that also measure humidity levels. For a very small fee, this allows you to easily monitor the air quality in your home.

If you find there is too much humidity or if you are located near a body of water or maritime area, there are effective solutions to dehumidify the air. To do this, choose an electric dehumidifier that will be efficient and will not pose a health risk. Some chemical dehumidifiers may contain products that are toxic and are relatively ineffective in comparison. The volume of air treated by electric models, often equipped with Pelletier cooling, is even greater because they are equipped with a fan to circulate the air in the room. Additionally, they have the advantage of having air filters that reduce the presence of bacteria in the air.

If you or your partner are prone to snoring and complicate each other's night, you can try sprays containing seawater. These clean the nostrils, improve the oxygenation of the body during sleep, and reduce the risk of snoring. There are also effective anti-snoring dentures called dental orthotics. Consult your dentist in order to be fitted correctly for a pair. A poorly adapted or poor-quality denture could create dental problems that are best avoided.

Brightness can also disturb your sleep. Ineffective or sometimes nonexistent shutters can interfere with your sleep if there is nearby lighting. If you are exposed to bright lights at night or sunlight too early, it can produce a natural alarm that may not be ideal for your schedule or if you wake up easily. The technical solutions are simpler for this, since all you need are quality blackout curtains. Make sure you use fabrics that are perfectly opaque and will not let light through. It is recommended to place them as close as possible to the window and to make an overlapping margin on each side as wide as possible to block out all light.

Psychological Improvements

THIS IS CERTAINLY an issue you have started to work on. I can confirm its importance. It is essential to take the time and care daily to reduce the problems of everyday life and to solve the questions that seem invasive to you in your waking hours. Though this is a long-term work that will bring its fruits in improving the quality of your sleep, you can start more simple activities to support your ability to relax. We are sometimes subject to anxious phases, and this method will allow you to feel more balanced quickly, in many aspects of your life, as you adopt techniques.

Today, there are many ways to incorporate relaxation practices into your daily life. Relaxation is a means, but not the goal. The goal is a state of peace that can be more and more present in your life every day. Among the relaxation techniques you can use are different types of yoga and meditations. For these, take the time to find out what seems to be in line with your needs. There are extremely slow forms yoga as well as very dynamic varieties. Some are suitable for one type of person, but not all are suitable for everyone.

Regarding meditation techniques, try to find a place and practice that suits you, one for which you feel an affinity. Meditation techniques exist in most spiritual traditions and are also taught in nonsecular settings by different teachers and therapists. Be open—spending time in a place that is not directly related to your culture does not commit you to anything. Even if you find an experience does not correspond to your needs, you can always leave, having learned something, whether it was a new technique or the traditions of a different culture. The vast majority of places offering meditation are accustomed to welcoming people of different religions or cultures. Many centers offer times of meditation in a perfectly secular setting.

If it feels too foreign to you, or if you do not feel like you are in a moment of life to explore this type of place, you can simply create a beneficial habit. It can be a time for you to simply breathe, to pause, to feel a peaceful state settle in you. Or you can take a walk outside and immerse yourself in nature. This provides automatic healing for most of us. Take some time for yourself. You will see that ten or fifteen minutes per day is enough to allow you to find calm in your daily life.

You can also find time to relax and regenerate through wellness massages, reflexology, cranial-sacral therapy, and other types of bodywork.

The key idea is to make the moments of peace that you experience every day grow in frequency and depth. By focusing on this, little by little, you can begin to find solutions to your problems and improve your quality of life. With time and diligence, the daytime fog from sleepless nights will be definitively changed.

Stimulants and Sleep Deregulators

SENSITIVITY TO THE myriad of exciting things we find in our society (legal or not) depends entirely on the constitution of each individual. Each person will have a different response and tolerance to one substance or another. However, it is very likely that, regardless of your sensitivity to a product, it will disturb your sleep in some way.

In general, it is not recommended to drink caffeinated beverages seven to eight hours before falling asleep (have the last beverage before 4:00 p.m.). For some people, this will go beyond that. Energy drinks should be avoided if possible. Otherwise, stop drinking them before 2:00 p.m.

There is only one rule that is really worthwhile for everyone, and that is getting to know yourself and your body's responses over time. Feel free to keep a small logbook. Noting your habits over the course of several weeks is an important and often insightful exercise. You can also note the times of the various stimulants you have used, the quality of sleep you have, and the sensation you feel after waking up.

The various so-called "light" drugs, such as tobacco, alcohol, and marijuana significantly alter your quality of sleep. Although for some people this may make it easier to fall asleep at first, there is a high chance that even a slight addiction, psychological or physical, can shift your sleep rhythm. The best way is to be able to honestly describe the various substances you consume. It is good for people who wake up frequently at night or who experience light sleep to know that smoking tobacco and/or drinking alcohol before bedtime increases the risk of both.

Here I must note a special warning. Among all the somewhat magical and instant solutions available in pharmacies, sleeping pills and barbiturates certainly have more defects than virtues. If you have already tried them, you probably have noticed that even if they can help you fall asleep, waking up is not only difficult but often accompanied by a feeling of heaviness and a much more intense fog than usual that lasts throughout the day. Homeopathic pills, at least all the ones I've tried, also have this effect, although less so.

We have seen together that, more often than not, insomnia is caused by a disorder or imbalance that has likely deregulated your rhythm. If, thanks to these pills it may be possible for you to fall asleep earlier for a few nights, their effect is not guaranteed. Many nights of insomnia are usually experienced despite their intake. What is certain, however, is that the next day will be difficult because they only allow a very poor, artificial sleep. If you have become accustomed to using them and you still do not feel closer to a solution to your problems, put them aside. If they were prescribed for you, ask your doctor for advice. It may be necessary to reduce the dosage or change the treatment before you can safely stop taking them. If you are hesitant to take them, I would advise you not to use them unless explicitly prescribed by your doctor or specialist, as they do nothing to heal the underlying conditions often associated with insomnia. They only mask the symptoms. In any case, be careful to avoid self-medication by using one substance or another, as this could have disastrous consequences on your health.

It is not always easy to get free of certain addictions. That is why it is imperative to observe, in order to become aware of their effects on your psychological and physical state. Getting to know yourself and developing an honest awareness of how you work will make it much easier for you to make the right choices.

I invite you to keep a small notebook or to take notes on your phone to record the hour and minute, each time you consume a substance you know acts as a stimulant or deregulator. You will see that this simple exercise can help you to regulate your substance intake more appropriately, as it allows you to observe concretely the relationship between the consumption of different substances and the time you fall asleep and/or the quality of your sleep. Then, with data in hand, you can act effectively.

Perform a few tests: change a habit that you think maybe disturbing your sleep. For example, instead of having your last coffee at 5:30 p.m., limit it to 3:30 p.m. for a week and note any changes at the end of the seven days. If you are used to drinking a bit of alcohol in the evening, try not to drink at all or stop drinking seven hours before bedtime. Observe the effects this may have on your sleep or mood. Make clear notes that allow you to follow your habits.

Sometimes, it may seem difficult or even impossible to stop certain habits. Don't worry; you don't need to make a jarring or dramatic change right away. A relatively easy way to start practicing self-discipline is by setting up a time limit after which you stop drinking. Remember what's at stake: the possibility of a real night's sleep.

To keep it simple in the beginning, it's important you don't feel like you are depriving yourself too much of something. Just be disciplined and perfectly honest with yourself when taking notes. There will be no one there to judge you; the observations you make are for you and only available to you. You can either destroy them or keep them once the exercise is completed, whichever feels right. This exercise is just a matter of observing and developing a clear awareness of your current situation and all the factors that can be hindering your healing. Little by little, you will be able to find a healthy rhythm that corresponds to your lifestyle and does not feel like a deprivation, but on the contrary, a liberation.

Chapter 4

Studying Your Sleep Rhythm

THE FIRST STEP toward change, as in many processes, is to make an assessment in order to understand the dysfunctions for which you are trying to find solutions. A graph provides a clear and convenient representation of a complex set of factors. This is the case for insomnia. It is sometimes surprising to see how simply writing your observations and graphically representing them for study provokes awareness that can be an important step toward improvement.

When I went to see a psychologist, he recommended this exercise to me. After looking at the data, it was clear that my daily rhythm of sleeping and waking up was completely chaotic, though I was not in an acute phase of insomnia. I would go to bed at 11 p.m. one night and 2 a.m. or sometimes even 3 a.m. the next. Sometimes I would fall asleep at 10 p.m., thinking it was perfect because I would finally be able to recover a few hours of sleep, but never before had I considered the image of my bedtime rhythm as a whole.

The technique is extremely simple. On a sheet of paper, write a calendar for the next two weeks. Upon rising, write down the approximate time you fell asleep, the time you woke up, and note from one to five the quality of sleep: one for a very bad night to five for a perfect one.

The graphs were created with the intention to be functional for the largest number of people. They are based on a conventional work schedule. The hours displayed on the vertical axis in the upper quadrant allow for a wide range of bed times. Wake-up hours are displayed in the lower quadrant. They are designed to be able to work for people who go to bed very early in the evening as well as for those who go to bed very late at night.

You can download a printable PDF version or high definition pictures of the graphs here :

https://www.booksforachange.com/free-sleep-evaluation-tools/

Keep this sheet near your bed where you will see it every day, to help yourself remember to record your data. For two weeks, record your rhythm every day. Then add your notes about the hours you consumed products (coffee, alcohol, drugs, tobacco, medication) that could have impacted your sleep.

Below is a blank example that you can use (fig. 1).

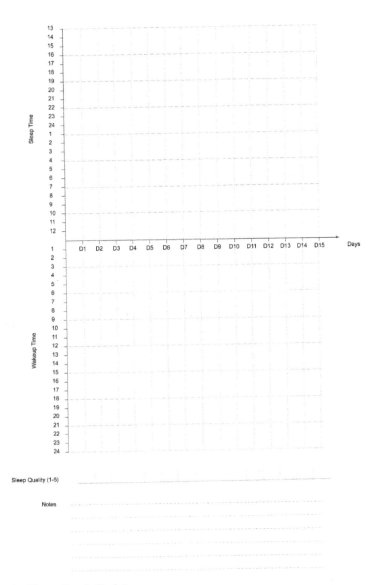

Fig. 1 - Sleep Graph Skeleton
https://www.booksforachange.com/free-sleep-evaluation-tools/

This exercise gives you an excellent visual representation of your sleep rhythm and can help you clearly detect any irregularities or bad habits.

If your habits are good, as in the example below (fig. 2), this curve should be relatively linear during the week and may have a slight variation over the weekend. Though it is tempting, keep in mind that the ideal is to avoid compensating for a lack of sleep on weekends.

If you observe significant changes between the different days of the week, as in the graph below (fig. 3), it is highly likely that a disturbed sleep rhythm is a major contributing factor to your insomnia.

Through recording your habits graphically, you will be able to visually understand that to have a good sleep rhythm, it is important to be consistent with the time you go to bed and the time you wake up.

Sometimes, having a partner makes it much easier to regulate yourself than if you were alone. On the other hand, for light sleepers, having someone at their side can be a difficulty. If this is the case, calmly speak about the different things that can be improved with your partner. If necessary, suggest sleeping separately from time to time when sleep difficulties are severe.

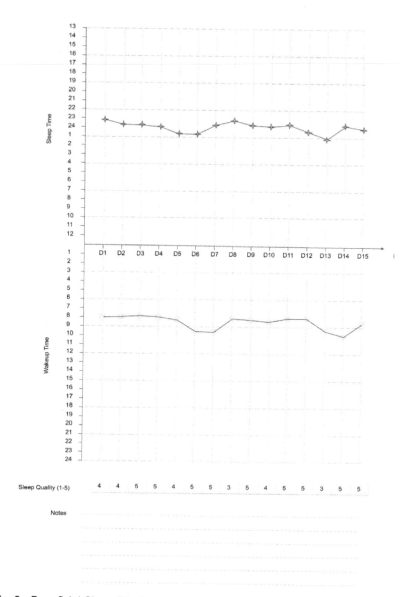

Fig. 2 - Beneficial Sleep Rhythm
https://www.booksforachange.com/free-sleep-evaluation-tools/

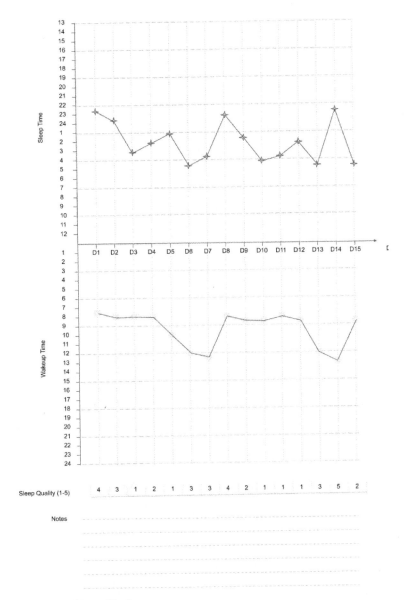

Fig. 3 - Broken Sleep Rhythm
https://www.booksforachange.com/free-sleep-evaluation-tools/

CHAPTER 5

What Are Your Sleep Needs?

ON THE SUBJECT of sleep, not all of us are equal. Some will have a physiological need for long nights, while others can feel rested after just a few hours of sleep. However, many studies show that having less than seven hours of sleep does not allow the body and brain to perform necessary detoxification and repair processes. Spending a significant number of nights with less than seven hours, combined with a feeling of lack of sleep, creates significant risks for the body in the long term [9].

Recent studies conducted by the National Sleep Institute show that our need for sleep diminishes with age. For example, the recommended number of hours of sleep for newborns is between fourteen and seventeen hours. As soon as we hit nine years old, this amount decreases to between eleven and fourteen hours and continues to fall to between eight and ten hours for a teenager. Adults generally have a lower sleep requirement, which is between seven and nine hours. In discussions with health professionals, it is thought that this may be due in part to the decreasing need for the brain to record new information.

Note that the quality of sleep is equally important as duration. As you probably know, we sleep in a series of cycles. INSERM (The National Public Research Organization in France) defines the need for a good night's sleep as having between three and five sleep cycles of ninety minutes each for an adult.

The exercise in the previous chapter will allow you to assess the minimum number of hours of sleep you need to feel well rested. All you have to do is average the number of hours of sleep over a period of about two weeks to get an idea of your sleep needs. This is the amount you should aim for on a regular basis each night. Since it depends on your age, it is subject to change over the years.

After you have calculated the average number of hours you need, try to adopt a regular rhythm. In other words, try to stop your activities and go to bed at the same time and wake up around the same time every morning. This is a very important step in bettering the quality of your sleep in the long term. Improving this regularity is central, as it will act on the sleep signals your brain sends to your body.

You can proceed in stages. Start by trying to go to bed at the same time every night for one week. Though you may not feel the benefits during the first few days while your body adjusts to this new rhythm, noticeable improvements will be quick to come. Try to proceed one week at a time. The difference you will see in the following weeks will encourage you to adopt these changes for the long term. Afterward, make a goal to maintain this rhythm for one month. Gradually you will see that these changes will naturally integrate into your life according to your needs.

If you have been in a difficult phase of sleep, with little rest for several days, weeks, or months, keep in mind that the short-term and long-term objectives are different. In the short term, we may feel like we have an immediate need to rest in order to best face a difficult emotional situation. Maybe we must solve an important problem in the workplace or in our personal relationships. However, it is important to keep in mind that improving the quality of your sleep is a gradual process and that you should plan your actions by first considering their long-term results. This will lead you to a gradual improvement in the overall quality of your life. It is this direction that must be targeted beyond the search for an immediate solution. You will find in the rest of this book many tips that will allow you to act wisely and effectively, to better understand the situation you are in.

If this seems difficult for you, don't rush; there's no need to put pressure on yourself. You will see that, on the contrary, it will be by simply finding a natural state of relaxation that you will be able to regulate your rhythm again. You will wake up each day with more than enough energy to fully participate in the duties and joys of everyday life.

Also, among the events that allow us to set the rhythm of our daily lives, mealtimes are particularly important. Try to align your mealtimes, especially dinner, in a way that supports your rhythm in the healthiest way possible. Having dinner too late in the evening can delay your ability to fall asleep or even prevent you from sleeping entirely. Eating too much, too heavy, or too much fat can also have the same effects. In general, it is good to leave at least two hours between the end of the meal and the time you go to bed. Not only is this consideration conducive to sleep, it can also improve digestion, since lying down right after eating can increase the likelihood of gastric reflux and heartburn. Most importantly, however, eating early will allow you time to properly wind down and find a state of calm before going to sleep. This is the closing moment of your day, and it must also be part of the rhythm to be integrated into your daily life.

CHAPTER 6

Adopting Healthy Habits

THERE ARE TWO important states that the body functions in. One is the state where it will respond to the demands of the outside environment, to stressful situations. This corresponds to our active state, where the body breaks down and consumes the resources it needs to function throughout the day. The other is a state of rest, during which it can regenerate, assimilate, repair, and evacuate toxins. Interestingly, states of exhaustion are actually states of depletion, meaning the body has not been able to regenerate the resources it needs. In fact, repeated sleep deprivation in adolescents has been correlated with a smaller volume of brain mass. Poor-quality sleep over the years will gradually damage the vital systems and functions of the body.

This is why it is so important to change direction and move toward a long-term improvement in your sleep, for the care of your body as well as your psyche.

Anything that aids you to relax and follows the guidelines of healthy sleep habits, without taking drugs or chemicals, is a good thing. It can be a shower or a hot bath, herbal tea, reading a book, or receiving a massage from your partner. Creating a favorable atmosphere, taking quiet time, or breathing a scent you like can help you to create a moment of relaxation.

An essential piece of advice concerns one of the most pervasive sources of sleep disturbance in our time: artificial light. Both ambient light and screen use before going to bed can greatly disrupt your sleep patterns.

Sleep is triggered by the natural cycle of the sun. It is the natural exposure to sunlight in the morning and then darkness at night that dictates the process our bodies use to regulate sleep, wake, and eat cycles. The progressive reduction of light in the evening acts as an external cue for the body to gradually plunge into the darkness of sleep. When the brain detects sunlight, this triggers reactions within the body that wake us up and boost our energy levels. However, different tones of light produce different effects. It is necessary to be particularly attentive to your exposure to cold, blue-toned lights.

The color temperature of a light source is expressed in degrees Kelvin (K). The colder the light, the higher the temperature. A temperature of 6500K corresponds to natural light around noon on a clear (not cloudy) day, and a temperature of 2800K to 3200K corresponds to sunset.

Generally, it is best to opt for warm indoor lights: 3000 to 4000 Kelvin. If you have mainly cold lights (bluish tones) in your home, avoid using them before bedtime and consider replacing them with warmer light sources.

In addition to the color temperature, try to get into the habit of turning down all ambient lighting at least thirty minutes before going to sleep.

Exposure to light emitted by screens before going to bed may be one of the main sources of difficulty falling asleep in modern life. This is now widely recognized, yet it still receives too little attention. So, try to avoid all screens—computers, smartphones, and others. It is the light intensity perceived by the pupil that cues the body to move into an active state. Although the light of a tiny phone screen may seem negligible, focusing your undivided attention directly on it causes your brain to perceive it as your main source of light. It is quite possible that by acting just on this point, you will quickly perceive a clear change and greater ease in regulating your sleep cycles. For example, choose to use an e-reader with a specially designed backlight, or choose a traditional book over reading on a telephone or tablet.

If you really must use your smartphone or tablet at night, establish good habits now by reducing the brightness of the screen to the minimum necessary. However, it is not advisable to continue surfing the internet, checking your emails, or reading the news. Select an activity that allows you to disconnect from your daily routine, like reading a novel that takes you to another time or to other latitudes. Maybe you would prefer to read a biography about someone who inspires you or any type of work that interests you and allows you to escape from everyday life for a few moments. This is an excellent option.

Later, we will see the importance of detaching yourself from everything that brings you back to negative, anxious thoughts; internal questioning; and an overly active use of your mind. You will surely notice that in the moments when you are completely relaxed, brilliant ideas tend to appear. Sometimes these ideas lead you to the resolution of a conflict that has been weighing on you, or at least important elements to solve it can arise.

This is logical. Thinking over and over about a subject that disturbs us during the day while operating in a state of tension limits our perspective and causes us to see an equally limited number of possible solutions. Once we are able to distance ourselves from the subject for a time and fully relax, the brain is able to create new associations between ideas. We enter a state that is naturally conducive to creativity. In the course of making these associations, new thoughts or ideas arise freely and allow us to consider new points of view and find creative solutions.

For many, evening is a time to take stock of the day. Do this before you lie down for bed, and be aware that once the light goes out, it's time to sleep. Resolve to leave all the day's business aside and rest.

The bed is a place to sleep or a place to make love. If you can't sleep, it's healthier to get up and go to another room to read. Return to bed half an hour to an hour later, or when you feel sleep approach.

In order to facilitate more regular nightly cycles, performing small "ceremonies" can be very effective. Consider bedtime as a time in and of itself. Think of all the calm and restful activities you would find enjoyable, or for some, this could even be a period of complete inactivity. For example, take time to take care of your plants, spend some quality time with your family, play a quiet game, or simply allow yourself to observe the quietness of the night coming. This time of day need not be particularly long; half an hour or three-quarters of an hour is more than enough. It is a time you can take for yourself that will prepare you for an excellent night of sleep.

Don't try to force yourself into thinking that you're going to succeed solving your insomnia forever in one night. It is healthier to move forward gradually, to be tolerant and gentle with yourself throughout this process, and to accept that it takes time. Once you begin to see the benefits these changes will bring, it will be easier for you to come back to them by integrating them into your daily routine.

CHAPTER 7

The Mechanisms of Falling Asleep

AFTER THE SUN sets, the brain sends a signal to the body through the hormonal system to trigger sleep. You've probably noticed that we naturally tend to synchronize our rhythm with the cycle of the sun when we spend time in nature. It is often surprising how easy it is to fall asleep after you have tuned into the simple rhythm of the countryside. The air is cleaner, and you can immerse yourself in a quiet environment. But the magic lies in the inner calm, the deceleration of our daily life that returning to a more natural tempo brings.

This is quite difficult to find in cities, where the pace of life is maintained by artificial light after sunset. Night becomes like a second day, where everything is designed to extend periods of activity. For thousands of years, communities were governed by the same phases of going to bed and waking up. Today, morning workers meet night workers in transport. This change is inevitable, and we need to adapt to it.

It is important to downplay the idea of sleep. You can compare it to nutrition. Just because you don't eat for a day doesn't mean you're going to die. Ideally, each meal should be balanced, but if you were unable to eat a couple of meals, your body would adapt and find sufficient resources to function properly. It is the same when you have had a bad night or two of sleep. Of course you will feel more tired the next day, but during the following nights, your body will readjust itself automatically.

One of the important laws of physiology called *homeostasis* is described as follows:

Higher living beings are an open system with many relationships with the environment. Changes in the environment trigger reactions in the system or affect it directly, leading to internal system disturbances. Such disturbances are normally kept within narrow limits because automatic adjustments within the system come into action, and, in this way, large oscillations are avoided, while internal conditions are kept more or less constant [...]. The coordinated physiological reactions that maintain most of the body's dynamic equilibrium are so complex and unique to living organisms that it has been suggested that a particular designation be used for these reactions: homeostasis [10].

In other words, if an organism is subject to stress due to its environment, it will automatically seek to regain its own balance once the source of the stress has disappeared.

That implies two things.

The first is that you have every chance of finding a solution to your insomnia. So there is no reason to ask extreme questions such as whether you are at risk of dying from prolonged sleep deprivation. As long as there is no one physically jumping on you all the time to keep you awake, it is not fatal. If insomnia is produced by an internal condition, your body will try to rebalance itself, and sooner or later, you will end up sleeping.

The second is that from the moment you put your finger on what causes this internal stress (pain, anxiety, disruptive emotions, drug or alcohol use, medication, nightlife) and you begin to address the problem, you will automatically recover sleep, and your insomnia will disappear.

The main change we are going to make together is in our relationship with sleep. We're going to empower ourselves and use this time of night, this time of rest, to your advantage. To do this, we must avoid entering into negative thought patterns when we are impatient and waiting for sleep. This only ends up making us feel desperate when sleep does not come.

We have to realize that it is the fact that we keep problems running over and over in our minds that often prevents us from falling asleep and creates a vicious circle. Poor sleep makes us more irritable the next day. This makes it difficult to make good decisions and for us to feel fully in line with ourselves. We then tend to create new problems—which, in other circumstances, would usually be avoided—rather than finding solutions.

The decision to leave problems aside in order to breathe and regain the pleasure of living is already the most effective way to start solving the issues that affect you. After doing this, you can gradually develop an entirely different attitude. The time you spend in your bed will truly become a time of rest. When sleep takes a long time to come, think back to the analogy with food and remember that even though you may be a little tired the next day, everything will be fine. At worst, you'll recover the next night. By learning to accept the situation and to find peace, you put all the chances of falling asleep on your side. So, enjoy the time, and above all, relax.

We have everything to gain by staying as relaxed as possible. As we have seen, when you enter into a state of true relaxation, the body begins to go into a phase of recovery. It begins the restoration process of all the internal systems that will allow you to find the necessary energy the next day.

CHAPTER 8

Introduction to the Method

THIS METHOD IS the result of three major understandings that have occurred at different times in my life. I have understood their complementarity over the past few years, before I could definitively develop this technique and judge its effectiveness. This book is the culmination and distillation of what I have learned, and I hope it will benefit as many people as possible.

First, we have to state the importance of relaxing the body and mind while entering into the sleep phase. Indeed, it is very difficult to fall asleep in a state of stress or tension. When you try, falling asleep is often delayed, and you usually wake up multiple times during the night. You already know this without needing me to detail it too much. It is very interesting to observe that the rhythm of the breath has a significant effect on our ability to relax. It also helps to regulate the heart rate.

You have probably noticed that physical tensions in the body are quite different from one day to the next and are highly dependent on our emotional state. Some days, when you go to bed, you may feel nervous, some days excited, and some days tranquil. Depending on our moment of life and the particular day, our emotional and physical condition in the evening varies. It is therefore important to understand that to facilitate falling asleep, the body and mind must enter a state of deep relaxation.

It is not a question of setting a goal or putting pressure on yourself to relax. This would seem absurd! Start to see relaxation and rest in a different light: it is both a pleasure and a need. It is your time.

Learning to relax is a practice, and like any practice, it requires a level of self-discipline. You must choose whether you want to rest or stay active. When you start to relax, you can decide whether you want to return to thoughts that invade you, or you can make a strong decision to leave these thoughts aside and accept real rest.

Try to stay on course. It is perfectly normal for us to drift sometimes, but put the helm in the correct direction right away. Do this without tension and without the objective of producing a result. Simply enjoy the time to rest. The recovery you are looking for is in this relaxation already. This time is yours. It is entering into a positive state of mind and applying the relaxation techniques that will allow us to find serenity and dissipate the different tensions we all accumulate over the course of our day.

The second important idea is the one we have just discussed in the previous chapter: the signal the brain transmits to the whole body to let it know that it is time to sleep. It happens when the brain understands that the day is over and there is nothing left to do. It is essential to understand this role as a catalyst. Sometimes it is triggered by an unconscious, automatic process, such as the observation of a change in the environment—for example, observing a decrease in light or a decrease in stimuli. However, choosing to ask yourself the question, "Is there anything I still need to do, or is my day over?" is a conscious decision that can trigger unconscious signals to the body that either facilitate sleep or keep you active. It is an essential step to take before going to bed. As long as you know and accept that your day is complete, sleep can be triggered.

If you still need or want to do things, then the role of the brain is to keep us awake in order to solve the problems of everyday life. As we are conditioned to operate in a hyperactive society, it is often in this stage that we have difficulty accepting that we need to slow down. However, this is the crucial moment that we must choose to stop thinking about work, scrolling through social media, and/or answering emails and try to put our body and mind at ease. This is how we can be much more effective the next day.

This brings us to the main idea: as long as the mind has control over our thoughts, we continually return to loops of reflection and analysis. We try to deal with situations in a future that does not exist, or we go back to situations in the past that we can never return to. We often recount situations from the events of the day or of past days—the conflicts, disagreements, or stressful situations for which we feel we must find an answer. This generates a state of tension in the body that can result in annoyance, boredom, feelings of anger, anxiety, or others that will prevent sleep.

I have practiced meditation for several years and have participated in sessions where the goal was to keep the mind calm and free of thoughts. At some point or another, every practitioner encounters the same difficulty: staying awake.

It is especially difficult in the afternoon after a large meal, but the struggle to stay awake is inevitable, regardless of the time of day. Even after several days of sitting in meditation, managing not to fall asleep in broad daylight, in a seated position, is really a challenge in itself. Indeed, when the brain has no thought to chew on, no memory to revisit, and no past or future situation to imagine, it then has only one desire: falling asleep.

When I was still experiencing insomnia, I applied this advice, and it permitted me to find more tranquility in my life, have a much better rhythm, and experience greater ease in falling asleep. This was a major accomplishment for me at that time. Yet, despite the notable improvements, I was still too often confronted with the same problem: I would be very close to putting myself and all of my thoughts to sleep. Then, as I felt the wave of sleep approach, my thoughts would take their threads back. I would all but lose the possibility of finding sleep again and would often end up maintaining a semi-awake state in my bed.

After I understood this principle of how the brain works, I was able to incorporate it into my method and obtain a complete technique that works almost every time. I was thirty-five years old when I finally reached my goal of sleeping soundly every single night. Today I am forty-one. It is now possible for me to fall asleep effortlessly when I want. Sometimes it may still take me a bit of time to fall asleep, but it usually doesn't exceed half an hour. Since most of my life I always needed four to five hours just to fall asleep, this was cause for celebration.

There are still times when I have difficulty falling asleep because of a problem I experienced during the day. But these nights can be counted on the fingers of one hand, over the course of a year. In parallel with these changes, there was a clear improvement in my quality of life, and my levels of anxiety were profoundly reduced.

As soon as I feel that the night may be more difficult, I use this method and take particular care with the relaxation process. I know that if I am self-disciplined, any difficulties will dissipate. I know that I will easily be able to have quality rest every single night.

Chapter 9

The Method: Step by Step

Preliminaries

AS WE SAW in the previous chapter, we will begin the journey back to sleep by preparing for bedtime. First, decide what time you want to fall asleep, and allow yourself forty-five minutes beforehand to begin winding down. Though this time can be reduced once your sleep cycles improve, it is best to always leave yourself a minimum of half an hour. This is a time dedicated to an activity that you enjoy, that interests you, and that makes you feel good. Again, giving yourself this time to relax is very important. It acts as a decompression chamber between day and night, where you can change pace and move on to a time of rest.

Next, it's good to think about what you can change in your room to improve your quality of sleep. Perhaps it is a good day to put fresh sheets on your bed to create a sense of well-being or take the opportunity to open the windows wide and allow fresh air to fill the room. Keep your bedroom cool when you go to bed. The warming process of the body, when lying down, helps us to fall asleep. Remember that the ideal bedroom temperature is 65° F (18° C).

Before you begin the activity you have chosen, take great care to ensure that the general lighting is dimmed. Try to set aside all digital devices with a display screen, or if you need to use them momentarily, adjust the brightness accordingly. Use the minimum amount of light necessary for your activity, turn off all unnecessary or overly bright lights, and try to avoid exposing yourself to any direct lighting. This, as we have seen, is very important because it will help synchronize the hormonal signals sent from your brain to the rest of your body.

❊ ❊ ❊

If you tend to overthink at night:

Most people do, so don't worry. It is important to understand that one of the most important things to do to find sleep easily is to accept that change often occurs gradually. This helps us to put aside any frustration and is especially true if we are to succeed in reducing the flow of thoughts and questions that can overwhelm us. A wise philosopher summed it up with this sentence: "It is not by walking on the caterpillar that you get a butterfly."

It is easy to understand that good rest contributes to good decisions the next day. In this way, you have to be willing to break with the habits that are detrimental to you. From the moment you begin your time of relaxation, it should mean the end of reflections on topics related to your concerns. It's no longer time to try to solve problems or dwell on an issue that worries you, but time to enjoy your moment off.

To do this, we must respect a golden rule: accept, with

strong determination, to stop thinking about subjects that may cause anxiety, negative thoughts, or issues that have worried you during your day. This does not mean that thoughts will suddenly cease to pop up in your mind, but that you should try not to get into a fight with or a further reflection about any of them. It is much simpler to let go. You must deeply accept that these issues are no longer relevant in the evenings, when you have chosen to go to bed. You can leave these thoughts aside for tonight and come back to them tomorrow with a clear and lucid mind. For now, when they come to you, try to simply acknowledge them and let them go.

So, what should you replace these reflections with?

The pleasure of living, of finding peace and quiet, and all the things that interest you deeply and for which you may not have had time anymore. If you find it difficult to leave troubling topics aside, you can ask yourself the following question: "Even if I could find an answer to these questions, would the world fundamentally change for me?" It is likely that a few days or weeks later, new questions or problems would arise that cause you stress or anxiety in the same way.

These life problems are normal and recurrent, but they must not invade your nights and disturb your rest. Imagine what you would do if you saw a child close to danger: you would act immediately to put a safe distance between the child and whatever the danger was. In the same manner, you must define the right boundary for the thoughts that affect you at night. This limit lies in the time when you are active, the daytime. If habits push you to carry these thoughts close to you at night, act as if you are taking care of a child who does not see the danger. Our role is to say stop for our own well-being.

You have the possibility, in this very moment, to change your relationship to the world by relaxing, enjoying being present, breathing, and living this small moment before sleep, not in stress but in the pleasure of being alive. Can you enjoy a good meal if you only have five minutes to eat and have to solve a dispute at the same time? You appreciate rest when you know how to give yourself the time to rest.

We have to get out of this old way. You'll find that by doing this, you open up space that will allow you to truly enjoy life.

Take the time to think about the beautiful side of the world, and if sometimes it's hard to see, remember that there are so many things to be grateful for! Think of nature, its strength and beauty, the different qualities you appreciate in the people around you, the pleasure of meeting someone new, the connection with a pet, the taste of your favorite fruit, the scent of wood or freshly cut grass, of a wildflower. Think of that feeling when you are on the beach, listening to the rhythm of the waves; in the peace and quiet of a forest; in the bath or watching the stars on a warm summer night.

※ ※ ※

If you feel the need to take stock of your day:

If you wish and feel the need, you can start by making time to take stock of your day before beginning your relaxing activity. It is important, however, that this moment of introspection be of a limited duration. Set a time in advance, and try to stick to it. If you think you might get lost in thought, you can put a reminder on your phone. Time has to become a friend again, and for that you need to keep a moment of relaxation that is just for you.

You can think back to the bright moments of your day, the difficulties you may have encountered, as well as possible solutions to any unresolved issues. We all experience complications in the course of our days; this is inherent to the human condition. While it is important not to avoid them, it is equally important to know how to move on to other things. End your retrospection on a positive aspect of the day. It may be the progress you have made on a project or the good conversations you have had with others. It can even be something simple like a good meal, a place you have enjoyed or the smile of a child you have seen. Before you finish, save a minute or two for your conclusion. Ideally, you can devote fifteen to twenty minutes to it and then close this reflection and move on to the relaxation.

When the time for these reflections is over, be at peace. You now know that you have devoted the right amount of time to it. If you were able to make progress on certain points, that's great. If this time allowed you to simply revisit your day, that's fine too. As the saying goes, "night is the best time for advice."

You'll see more clearly tomorrow when you've rested. So far, you've done what you needed to do. Now it's time to take care of yourself in order to have a great day tomorrow.

※ ※ ※

Move on to a relaxing activity:

It's time to take some time for yourself. You can prepare a hot bath or shower and then immerse yourself in a novel. Choose literature that doesn't bring you back to large dilemmas or social issues. Of course, there is no question of avoiding these subjects in your life, but if you want to do your best for the world around you, you need to start by taking care of yourself and your ability to sleep. Once you restore your energy and feel balanced and able to rest, you can then work effectively on these larger subjects. Right now your mind needs to be able to turn to horizons of calm and peace.

This can be a great opportunity to reconnect with your passions and find books on these subjects, to reconnect with pieces of art, to dive into a comic book, or to do a manual craft like knitting. If you feel particularly stressed, I would advise you to create a relaxing moment for yourself, take a bath, or give yourself permission to just enjoy being calm and disconnected from the world. If you live as a couple or in cohabitation, you can propose the exchange of a massage, invent a story together, or play a short game. Avoid games that could lead to frustration; keep it light. For the moment, leave aside all activities that require deep learning and reflection. The goal is not to stimulate the mind but to wind down.

Again, when it's time to go to bed, make sure you use low light in the hallways and in your bedroom. It is very important to maintain low lighting until you go to sleep.

Step 1 - Decide if It Is Time to Sleep

ONCE YOU GO to bed with the lights off, the first question to ask yourself, strange as it may seem, is "Do I really want to sleep?"

We may want to sleep in order to feel rested, but there are times, if we dig a bit deeper into what we would truly like to do, we find that we want to stay awake and continue to read or to wonder what we want to do the next day, despite being tired. There is nothing wrong with that, but it is important not to do this in your bed. It's best to get up and continue this activity in another room. First, it will allow you to be clear with what you want and to finish what you have in mind if you need to. Furthermore, from now on, it is imperative that you dedicate the bedroom entirely to rest, sleep, and making love. This means that it will no longer be a place to question yourself or to go on with mental activities that are usually part of your daytime life. The bed is now exclusively the place where you go to sleep or to be with your partner.

After you have asked yourself this question and it is clear to you that your desire is to sleep, then it is time to begin the breathing exercise and a more specific relaxation technique that will lead you into sleep. We'll start with a simple relaxation of the body. To do this, you will take a series of twenty-one breaths. Breathe simply, calmly, and gently, without forcing anything. Simply follow your natural breathing pattern and count the number of breaths on the exhalation without losing the thread.

At first, this seemingly simple exercise may be much more difficult than you would think. It is perfectly normal for thoughts to come into your mind. Just let them slide aside. Don't get attached to any of them. Avoid entering into subjects that the mind suggests or into any deep contemplation. Just stay with your breath. Take a calm inhalation and an equally peaceful exhalation. Focus on the sensation of the air flowing in and out of your nostrils.

When you lose your breath count or realize that you have simply stopped counting, don't worry. Just go back to the beginning, starting with your next breath. If at first you can't hold your attention long enough to remember the number of the breath you are on, it's okay. With time and practice, it will get easier. Do this exercise for ten to fifteen minutes before moving on to the next one.

Don't make completing this exercise into a goal—something to be achieved. There's nothing to achieve. Think of this exercise as a time of self-care, a time for you. Each time you breathe deeply and serenely, your body relaxes more and more, making it easier to find your way back to yourself. Despite having practiced this technique for years, I frequently have to start the count over two or three times, even when my mind is clear.

Over time, it is easy to learn to appreciate how this breathing exercise can be deeply relaxing and nourishing. As you relax, you may notice that you become more acutely aware of your physical or mental state. If you feel the need to continue the practice longer than outlined in this book, then feel free to repeat the exercise once or twice more, starting from the beginning.

When your body begins to enter and remain in a state of relaxation and rest, it is no longer in a state where it consumes resources but in a state where it can regenerate itself, even without sleep. It is important to keep this in mind. There is the misconception that if you do not sleep, you cannot be rested. This incorrect thought pattern can lead to anxiety-provoking speculation. By understanding and accepting the proper functioning of our body, by seeing clearly that once we lie down in a state of relaxation, the body already begins to recover its capacities, we can start to appreciate the time spent before falling asleep in proper measure, honoring this time by making it ours again.

Step 2 - Trigger the Sleep Wave

THE SECOND QUESTION to ask yourself is "Did I do everything I wanted to do in my day, or are there still things I could and should do before I go to sleep?"

This is an extremely important question, so don't neglect it! It will make it possible for you to end your working day psychologically and therefore allow your brain to send the signal to the rest of the body that it is time to sleep.

If, in answer to this question, you see that there is a short task left to do, then it is much wiser to get up, take the time to finish it, and then go back to bed. If it is a time-consuming task, like a report that you should be writing that you are behind on, then it is wise to accept that you are probably not going to finish it tonight. It is something that belongs to the following day, when you will be much more efficient. Then you will be able to put all your energy into your work, and chances are, the result will be of a much higher quality.

If you have done everything you could do before bed, the brain can transmit the message to the rest of the body. If your body is sufficiently relaxed and unwound, and your mind is calm, you will be able to feel a wave of sleep coming over you and probably won't need to go any further. Just let yourself be carried away by it.

Step 3 - Keep Attuned to a Relaxed State

DESPITE GOOD PREPARATIONS, sometimes the accumulated energy in the body or other factors create complications in falling asleep. The following technique will help you to overcome this.

In the dark, and preferably while lying comfortably on your back, observe the tensions in your body, moving from the feet to the head. Sometimes we may retain too much energy in the legs, lower abdomen, solar plexus, or lungs, for example. Though this may not prevent you from getting sleep, it is good to spend a bit of time dedicated to relaxing these physical tensions.

After observing where excess energy or strain in the body lies, start to relax the body, part by part, from bottom to top, starting with the feet. You can spend a little extra time when you feel that a certain body part or area needs longer to let go, but try to do this without getting absorbed in trying to force something to happen. Spending thirty seconds, no more, of focus on a tense muscle, organ, or part of the body is sufficient. Avoid the trap of getting lost in observing a specific point.

Beginning with the lower body, bring your attention to the toes. Imagine all the muscles in the toes softening and letting go. Then move on to the soles of the feet and finally the whole foot. Breathe calmly before moving on to the calves. Allow the calves to relax in the same manner, then the knees, and then the thighs. Move up the body, little by little, to release the whole pelvis and belly. Feel the muscles of lower back let go and sink into the bed underneath you. Soften the lungs, and feel them expand. Continue to the solar plexus and midback. Breathe.

Feel the muscles in the shoulders release. Move on to the arms and the forearms. Then bring your awareness to your hands, including the fingers. Continue to the neck. Feel any stress in the muscles of the neck let go. Allow the jaw to drop so that you can move it a little from left to right without the upper and lower teeth touching to remove all the remaining tension from the day. Finally, let the muscles of the lips and cheeks soften, followed by the muscles in the eyes, eyebrows, and forehead, all the way to the top of the skull.

As you get used to working through this exercise, you may feel your limbs grow heavy. By being particularly attentive to any subtle sensations, you may be able to feel a vibration slowly propagating throughout your body that corresponds to the transition into sleep.

Once the body is perfectly relaxed, shift your concentration to your breath, and as in the previous exercise, begin to count your breath cycles. When thoughts enter your awareness, let them slide away, being swept along without invading you. If you observe that you have entered into a thought, into an inner discussion, and have lost count of the exhalations, don't worry. Repeat the exercise from the beginning, counting up to twenty-one breaths.

After the first cycle, continue this exercise but this time without counting, just being careful not to entertain any thoughts, no matter how interesting they may seem. When the brain no longer has thoughts to control, it will naturally go into sleep mode.

Conclusion

IF IT IS still particularly difficult for you to fall asleep after you have completed this method, or if you have returned to a state of energy that does not allow you to fall asleep, repeat the steps in the order of this chapter, beginning at the point where it seems most appropriate to you.

Little by little, you will find that you are able to get to sleep whenever you want through self-discipline, without being too hard on yourself. With the knowledge of this technique and by working to improve your sleep whenever possible, slowly, other problems will most likely decrease, and you should notice the improvement in your quality of life.

It may take a bit of practice at first, but soon you should find that you will be able to control the duration of your sleep and your ability to fall asleep much better.

You will also see that the moments you spend in bed before falling asleep are now part of your rest. Even if the previous exercises based on breathing cycles last for a long time, especially at the beginning, your quality of rest will quickly improve. If you are able to keep your body and mind in a state of relaxation, then you will soon see the changes take place.

Don't forget to indulge in your relaxation time. Use it as a time for yourself to simply enjoy the calm of the night.

Uncover New Ideas

A FRIEND ONCE told me that she often imagined herself playing Mario Kart in order to help herself fall asleep. She would visualize the video game's endlessly scrolling roads, and this would inevitably make her so tired that she would drift off before she realized it. It's an idea I never would have thought of! But why not? In the end, the goal is to imagine a place where you can be safe and where your thoughts have no hold.

The #SleepKeys feed exists on Twitter and Instagram to share your successes, as well as ideas and solutions that have worked for you. The hashtag #SleepCuts is available to share difficulties related to sleep disorders and to post about their causes.

Feel free to look at the different ideas published by other readers that you may be able to use or adapt. You will see how many people have experienced a similar situation and how we can create brilliant solutions together.

Also, you can post your questions and find the relevant topics of your interest on the   dedicated forum: https://www.booksforachange.com/sleep-insomnia-forum/

Twitter

@SleepCounselor

#SleepKeys

#SleepCuts

Instagram

@SleepCounselor

#SleepKeys

#SleepCuts

Note: *While social networks can be great communication tools, be especially careful to use them sparingly. Browse them during the day if you like them, and log out early in the evening, preferably before dinner. As with other substances, some people may have developed strong addictions to these networks.*

Chapter 10

Rough Nights

WHEN IT COMES to sleepless nights, consider changing your system of thinking. Understand that the number of hours of sleep are not the only factor in determining the restorative quality of sleep. You have probably already experienced this: waking up from a very long night of sleep feeling completely fatigued and waking up after much shorter nights feeling refreshed.

The rule is that when you effectively return your body to a state of rest and relaxation, this has a restorative effect, much like sleep. Even more, the fact that you can choose to do this consciously, that you have control over this ability, is extremely self-empowering. You are then able to reclaim your ability to regenerate. So, if there are nights that are still difficult for you, the most important thing is to manage to relax. Even if you only sleep two or three hours during the night, you will see that the next day, you will not be so tired. The next night will certainly be full and very restful.

It is important to avoid the vicious circle of frustration that generates stress through the fear of not being able to fall asleep. Take the hours you would spend in bed worrying and be constructive with this time, give it real quality, real value. If you can't sleep for one night, it's okay. Just take care of your breathing, and focus on relaxing your body completely. Avoid entertaining recurring ideas, deep introspection, and intense questioning. If you feel yourself falling into cycles of thought, at the very least, get up to deal with a point that is troubling you, and no longer begin these reflections while you are in bed. Be aware of the importance of maintaining a state of positivity in order to lead your body to a state of repair.

If the thoughts are too intrusive or it is particularly difficult for you to calm down, you can do some visualization exercises. You can, for example, take an imaginary walk; think about certain places where you feel good, at peace, and safe; or something you have seen on a trip that fascinated you. You will see over time that short nights with a real quality of relaxation are even better than nights of sleep that seem complete in regard to quantity of hours.

Chapter 11

Micro-Naps

WHEN I HAD difficulty finding enough momentum during the day to accomplish all the tasks I needed to, a psychologist advised me to try taking naps "à la Dali." The artistic genius and explorer of the dream world that Salvador Dali was led him to invent a simple technique that allowed him to regain the energy sufficient for his creative ardor by taking a micro-nap during the day.

To do this, he sat in an armchair, holding a heavy key at the limit of balance between the thumb and forefinger of his left hand. He would then place an upturned plate on the floor under the key. When he began to relax in his armchair and enter into a light sleep, the muscles in his hand would release their grip on the key, which would fall onto the plate. The sound of it gave him the signal that it was time to wake up.

The principle is simple. It is a matter of relaxing the body and mind to allow the shift from an active state, where the body consumes resources, to a state of rest, where it will begin to regenerate itself and make the resources it needs to move through the day. This technique works by causing you to wake up as soon as the body relaxes. The sound of the key allows you to avoid going too deep into a sleep cycle from which it is difficult to come out.

It takes a bit of time to master the art of the micro-nap, but it is an extremely interesting technique. You will see how a very short rest period can restore a large capacity of psychic and physical energy. This will enable you to approach the second part of the day with renewed dynamism and a clearer mind.

Moreover, people practicing yoga have probably noticed that the postures intended for complete relaxation, often practiced lying down for just a few minutes, allow you to regain quite a bit of zeal. These types of practices, when you have the opportunity to do them during the course of a day, contribute to improving both your physical and mental capacity. They can improve the regularity of your sleep by allowing you to recuperate without shifting your sleep cycle.

Beware, however, of long naps. Avoid going into a deep sleep, otherwise waking up can be particularly difficult, and your rhythm of falling asleep may shift as a result. It is sometimes necessary to sleep longer during the day, due to occasional overactivity or jet lag, but this need remains exceptional. Try to refrain from taking excessively long naps where you hope to recover sleep, as you risk unbalancing your sleep cycle in the medium and long term. It is also recommended not to take a nap after 3 p.m., so as not to affect your sleep rhythm at night.

The important thing is to grasp the idea of this technique that Salvador Dali invented. You can practice it in a classic lying position with the help of an alarm clock if you feel more comfortable. In general, a light sleep state lasts ten to fifteen minutes. For naps, as for nightly sleep, the time of falling asleep differs from one person to the next. For example, if you know that it takes about twenty to thirty minutes to relax before falling asleep during a nap, then you can set an alarm clock for forty minutes after you lie down. Most people need a much shorter period of time to fall asleep, but again, this varies greatly from person to person. With a bit of practice, micro-naps will help you improve your sleep and can be a huge help when you face intense workloads. They are a tool to help you recover the necessary energy and concentration for your day when needed.

CHAPTER 12

Achieve the Life Balance You Want

IT'S ALWAYS EASY to pick up bad habits or to get out of sync on a trip because of a change in your life or simply by having left good practices aside a little too long. This is why, from the first time you start following the different tips and the method in this book, you should take the time to write down the benefits or changes you observe, in a notebook or on the back of the sheet on which you have written down your sleep curve.

Don't be fooled—if you have adopted good habits for a period of time and then slip back into habits that are not conducive to sleep for one or more weeks, your sleep cycle will start to deregulate again. It is also possible that the techniques we have seen together become less effective if they lose their freshness in your mind and your motivation becomes dull. Try to maintain coherence and a good rhythm in your progress without having to be radical.

Repeated overactivity, very frequent use of alcohol or other substances, and periodic changes of pace are likely to send you back to the starting point. There is no need to submit to a strict asceticism, in which any failure to maintain it may cause you to return to your old rhythm or habits. However, for people who feel the need and motivation for a total and immediate change, this can be very good. The best thing to do is to make a commitment with yourself for at least three months. But this is by no means an obligation.

If you have sufficient self-discipline and are able to be conscious and honest with yourself about your rhythm and habits, you can continue with your present way of life and try to improve it as you go along. If you think this is the right way to integrate these changes, then make sure you also do small check-ins for a period of three months, every week, on

Sundays. Feel free to keep a logbook that you can fill out to describe the week you've had, and note your intentions for the week ahead. For example, for the following week: "Week 3: Decrease to a maximum of three coffees per day, end daytime activities at 10 p.m."

This method, when used occasionally, will give you short-term help but will not allow you to make a lasting change toward a better quality of life, which is most likely your deepest wish. It's not easy to change overnight. You must work to calmly develop self-discipline without becoming frustrated if you do not immediately see the radical change you may like. Habits change gradually with consistent action and conviction. It is human nature; you are not alone with these difficulties.

As with any self-work, you may need to regain courage, get remotivated, and start again. To stay motivated, it is great to be aware of what you have already managed to accomplish. The important thing is to use this method as regularly as possible in the beginning. You can try to function in cycles of several weeks or months, depending on your situation and your abilities. This will allow you to gradually improve the quality of your sleep, keeping in mind that it has a positive impact on your work and personal fulfillment, as well as on your social relationships. The goal must be to attain the life balance you wish for yourself and, in turn, for others.

Keep in mind the simple considerations that led you to start this work. Think of the improvements you've already made. Don't forget that the key objective is not only to be able to get back to a good night's sleep but a life in which you can be fully present.

Chapter 13

Improving Your Quality of Sleep Over Time

AS YOU CAN see, you have done the hardest part: recognizing the problem and taking the first step toward a solution. Try the different recommendations, and enjoy the benefits.

Seize the opportunity to improve your quality of life now, and apply the advice that speaks to your situation. Make time for yourself every night, for half an hour or a little longer, to relax and enjoy the moment before falling asleep. You now have tools that will gradually help you get to sleep. Be confident and know that you can relax, that sleep will come. Appreciate the quality of time found during all the stages of relaxation, this time that may have been lacking in your life, time that is now yours again. Remember that relaxation is already a source of rest. Honestly define the length of time you wish to commit to applying the necessary discipline by being firm yet understanding with yourself.

Over the weeks, you can repeat the exercise in chapter 4 of writing down your sleep and wake times and plotting them on a graph. This document will allow you to remember what your sleep rhythm and quality used to be and how it has changed with new habits. The good results that you will achieve will certainly be the most motivating element in order not to lose the practices you have implemented.

You have the keys you need to recover your ability to sleep deeply, feel rested every time you wake up, and improve your quality of life. I hope that the experiences I have had and passed on to you in the best possible way will be of benefit to you. Don't forget that sleep also reflects our waking, psychic state. It is therefore a clear invitation to improve the quality of our daily lives to the same extent. Work to have increasingly healthy and relaxed relationships with others. Try to resolve the various practical, philosophical, or spiritual questions that come before you in your daily life, in order to move toward an accomplished present. This is for our highest good and therefore for the benefit of our relatives and friends also. Nighttime can help us to better understand our psyche and our emotions; daytime is when we can act on the world, and for that we must start by acting on ourselves.

Did you like this book?

Thanks for choosing this book. I hope it brought you valuable knowledge and you start seeing improvements in your life that will grow with time.

If you liked this work, you can actively participate in its success by leaving a review on your bookseller's website. Your help is precious and contributes more than you could know in making this book visible to the greatest number of people who may need it.

Discover the Community of Readers

Official Website

Get access to free downloads, forums, and news:

http://www.booksforachange.com/

Share your experiences on the forum:

https://www.booksforachange.com/sleep-insomnia-forum/

Subscribe to the newsletter

https://www.booksforachange.com/news/

Twitter

Stay up to date with new articles: @SleepCounselor

#SleepKeys

#SleepCuts

Instagram

Find valuable advice and inspiration: @SleepCounselor

#SleepKeys

#SleepCuts

Notes

1. https://news.gallup.com/poll/166553/less-recommended-amount-sleep.aspx

2. https://www.thegoodbody.com/sleep-statistics/

3. https://www.thegoodbody.com/sleep-statistics/

4. https://www.healthline.com/health/sleep-deprivation/effects-on-body#1

5. https://www.sciencedaily.com/releases/2018/06/180605154114.htm

6. https://www.psychologytoday.com/us/blog/neuronarrative/201812/understanding-the-connection-between-sleep-and-anxiety

7. https://www.webmd.com/sleep-disorders/guide/insomnia-symptoms-and-causes#1

8. https://www.ncbi.nlm.nih.gov/pmc/articles/PMC3181635/

9. https://www.ncbi.nlm.nih.gov/pmc/articles/PMC4651462/

10. Cannon B. Walter, (1932). The Wisdom of the Body. New York: W. W. Norton.